# This Book BELONGS TO

_____
_____

# Contact Details

_____
_____
_____
_____

Date: _____  Patient name: _____
APPOINTMENT: _____

Patient Details
_____
_____
_____
_____

Patient History
_____
_____
_____
_____

| SYMPTOMS | MEDICATION | CONCERNS |
|---|---|---|
|  |  |  |

My Thoughts and Notes
_____
_____
_____
_____
_____

Future Check Up/s
_____
_____
_____

IMPORTANT
_____
_____
_____

**Date:** _____  **Patient name:** _____

APPOINTMENT: _____

*Patient Details*
_____
_____
_____
_____

*Patient History*
_____
_____
_____
_____

| SYMPTOMS | MEDICATION | CONCERNS |
|---|---|---|
| | | |

*My Thoughts and Notes* — *Future Check Up/s*

_____  _____
_____  _____
_____  _____
_____  _____
_____
_____

IMPORTANT
_____
_____

Date: _____  Patient name: _____

APPOINTMENT: _____

## Patient Details
_____
_____
_____
_____

## Patient History
_____
_____
_____
_____

| SYMPTOMS | MEDICATION | CONCERNS |
|---|---|---|
|  |  |  |

### My Thoughts and Notes
_____
_____
_____
_____
_____

### Future Check Up/s
_____
_____
_____

### IMPORTANT
_____
_____

Date: _____  Patient name: _____

APPOINTMENT: _____

### Patient Details
_____
_____
_____
_____

### Patient History
_____
_____
_____
_____

| SYMPTOMS | MEDICATION | CONCERNS |
|---|---|---|
|  |  |  |

### My thoughts and Notes
_____
_____
_____
_____
_____

### Future Check Up/s
_____
_____
_____

IMPORTANT

Date: _____  Patient name: _____
APPOINTMENT: _____

## Patient Details
_____
_____
_____
_____

## Patient History
_____
_____
_____
_____

| SYMPTOMS | MEDICATION | CONCERNS |
|---|---|---|
|  |  |  |

## My Thoughts and Notes
_____
_____
_____
_____
_____

## Future Check Up/s
_____
_____
_____

IMPORTANT
_____
_____
_____

*Date:* _____  *Patient name:* _____

APPOINTMENT: _____

*Patient Details*

_____
_____
_____
_____

*Patient History*

_____
_____
_____
_____
_____

| SYMPTOMS | MEDICATION | CONCERNS |
|---|---|---|
|  |  |  |

*My Thoughts and Notes* | *Future Check Up/s*

IMPORTANT

**Date:** _____  **Patient name:** _____

APPOINTMENT: _____

## Patient Details
_____
_____
_____
_____

## Patient History
_____
_____
_____
_____

| SYMPTOMS | MEDICATION | CONCERNS |
|----------|------------|----------|
|          |            |          |

### My Thoughts and Notes
_____
_____
_____
_____

### Future Check Up/s
_____
_____
_____

### IMPORTANT
_____
_____

**Date:** _____  **Patient name:** _____

APPOINTMENT: _____

## Patient Details

_____
_____
_____
_____

## Patient History

_____
_____
_____
_____
_____

| SYMPTOMS | MEDICATION | CONCERNS |
|---|---|---|
|  |  |  |

### My Thoughts and Notes

_____
_____
_____
_____
_____
_____

### Future Check Up/s

_____
_____
_____

IMPORTANT

Date: _____  Patient name: _____
APPOINTMENT: _____

## Patient Details
_____
_____
_____
_____

## Patient History
_____
_____
_____
_____

| SYMPTOMS | MEDICATION | CONCERNS |
|---|---|---|
|  |  |  |

## My Thoughts and Notes
_____
_____
_____
_____
_____

## Future Check Up's
_____
_____
_____

IMPORTANT
_____
_____
_____

Date: _____  Patient name: _____

APPOINTMENT: _____

## Patient Details
_____
_____
_____
_____

## Patient History
_____
_____
_____
_____

| SYMPTOMS | MEDICATION | CONCERNS |
|---|---|---|
|  |  |  |

### My Thoughts and Notes
_____
_____
_____
_____

### Future Check Up/s
_____
_____
_____

### IMPORTANT
_____
_____

Date: _____ Patient name: _____

APPOINTMENT: _____

## Patient Details
_____
_____
_____
_____

## Patient History
_____
_____
_____
_____

| SYMPTOMS | MEDICATION | CONCERNS |
|---|---|---|
|  |  |  |

## My Thoughts and Notes
_____
_____
_____
_____
_____
_____

## Future Check Up/s
_____
_____
_____

IMPORTANT
_____
_____
_____

**Date:** _____  **Patient name:** _____

APPOINTMENT: _____

*Patient Details*
_____
_____
_____
_____

*Patient History*
_____
_____
_____
_____

| SYMPTOMS | MEDICATION | CONCERNS |
|---|---|---|
|  |  |  |

*My Thoughts and Notes* | *Future Check Up/s*

IMPORTANT

Date: _____  Patient name: _____

APPOINTMENT: _____

## Patient Details

_____
_____
_____
_____

## Patient History

_____
_____
_____
_____

| SYMPTOMS | MEDICATION | CONCERNS |
|---|---|---|
|  |  |  |

## My Thoughts and Notes

### Future Check Up/s

_____
_____
_____
_____
_____
_____

IMPORTANT

**Date:** _____ **Patient name:** _____

APPOINTMENT: _____

## Patient Details
_____
_____
_____
_____

## Patient History
_____
_____
_____
_____

| SYMPTOMS | MEDICATION | CONCERNS |
|----------|------------|----------|
|          |            |          |

## My Thoughts and Notes
_____
_____
_____
_____

## Future Check Up/s
_____
_____
_____

IMPORTANT
_____
_____

Date: _____  Patient name: _____

APPOINTMENT: _____

## Patient Details

_____
_____
_____
_____

## Patient History

_____
_____
_____
_____

| SYMPTOMS | MEDICATION | CONCERNS |
|---|---|---|
|  |  |  |

### My Thoughts and Notes

_____
_____
_____
_____
_____

### Future Check Up's

_____
_____
_____

IMPORTANT

_____
_____
_____

Date: _____ Patient name: _____
APPOINTMENT: _____

## Patient Details
_____
_____
_____
_____

## Patient History
_____
_____
_____
_____

| SYMPTOMS | MEDICATION | CONCERNS |
|---|---|---|
|  |  |  |

### My Thoughts and Notes
_____
_____
_____
_____

### Future Check Up/s
_____
_____
_____

IMPORTANT
_____
_____

*Date:* _____ *Patient name:* _____

APPOINTMENT: _____

*Patient Details*
_____
_____
_____
_____

*Patient History*
_____
_____
_____
_____

| SYMPTOMS | MEDICATION | CONCERNS |
|---|---|---|
|  |  |  |

*My thoughts and Notes*      *Future Check Up/s*

_____
_____
_____
_____
_____

IMPORTANT
_____
_____
_____

Date: _____  Patient name: _____

APPOINTMENT: _____

Patient Details
_____
_____
_____
_____

Patient History
_____
_____
_____
_____

| SYMPTOMS | MEDICATION | CONCERNS |
|---|---|---|
|  |  |  |

My Thoughts and Notes                    Future Check Up/s
_____        _____
_____        _____
_____        _____
_____
_____

IMPORTANT
_____
_____

*Date:* _____  *Patient name:* _____

APPOINTMENT: _____

*Patient Details*
_____
_____
_____
_____

*Patient History*
_____
_____
_____
_____

| SYMPTOMS | MEDICATION | CONCERNS |
|---|---|---|
|  |  |  |

*My Thoughts and Notes*     *Future Check Up's*

IMPORTANT

Date: _____    Patient name: _____

APPOINTMENT: _____

Patient Details
_____
_____
_____
_____

Patient History
_____
_____
_____
_____

| SYMPTOMS | MEDICATION | CONCERNS |
|---|---|---|
|  |  |  |

My Thoughts and Notes

Future Check Up/s

IMPORTANT

Date: _____ Patient name: _____

APPOINTMENT: _____

## Patient Details
_____
_____
_____
_____

## Patient History
_____
_____
_____
_____

| SYMPTOMS | MEDICATION | CONCERNS |
|---|---|---|
|  |  |  |

## My Thoughts and Notes
_____
_____
_____
_____
_____

## Future Check Up/s
_____
_____
_____

IMPORTANT
_____
_____
_____

Date: _____ Patient name: _____

APPOINTMENT: _____

### Patient Details
_____
_____
_____
_____

### Patient History
_____
_____
_____
_____

| SYMPTOMS | MEDICATION | CONCERNS |
|---|---|---|
|  |  |  |

### My thoughts and Notes
_____
_____
_____
_____
_____

### Future Check Up/s
_____
_____
_____

### IMPORTANT
_____
_____
_____

Date: _____   Patient name: _____

APPOINTMENT: _____

## Patient Details
_____
_____
_____
_____

## Patient History
_____
_____
_____
_____

| SYMPTOMS | MEDICATION | CONCERNS |
|---|---|---|
|  |  |  |

## My Thoughts and Notes
_____
_____
_____
_____
_____
_____

## Future Check Up/s
_____
_____
_____

IMPORTANT

Date: _____  Patient name: _____

APPOINTMENT: _____

## Patient Details

_____
_____
_____
_____

## Patient History

_____
_____
_____
_____

| SYMPTOMS | MEDICATION | CONCERNS |
|---|---|---|
|  |  |  |

### My Thoughts and Notes

_____
_____
_____
_____
_____
_____

### Future Check Up's

_____
_____
_____

IMPORTANT

Date: _____ Patient name: _____

APPOINTMENT: _____

Patient Details
_____
_____
_____
_____

Patient History
_____
_____
_____
_____

| SYMPTOMS | MEDICATION | CONCERNS |
|---|---|---|
|  |  |  |

My Thoughts and Notes

Future Check Up/s
_____
_____
_____

_____
_____
_____
_____

IMPORTANT
_____
_____

**Date:** _____  **Patient name:** _____

APPOINTMENT: _____

## Patient Details
_____
_____
_____
_____

## Patient History
_____
_____
_____
_____

| SYMPTOMS | MEDICATION | CONCERNS |
|---|---|---|
|  |  |  |

### My Thoughts and Notes
_____
_____
_____
_____

### Future Check Up/s
_____
_____
_____

IMPORTANT
_____
_____

Date: _____   Patient name: _____

APPOINTMENT: _____

Patient Details
_____
_____
_____
_____

Patient History
_____
_____
_____
_____

| SYMPTOMS | MEDICATION | CONCERNS |
|---|---|---|
|  |  |  |

My Thoughts and Notes · Future Check Up/s

IMPORTANT

Date: _____  Patient name: _____

APPOINTMENT: _____

## Patient Details

_____
_____
_____
_____

## Patient History

_____
_____
_____
_____

| SYMPTOMS | MEDICATION | CONCERNS |
|---|---|---|
|  |  |  |

## My thoughts and Notes

_____  
_____  
_____  
_____  
_____  

## Future Check Up/s

_____
_____
_____

IMPORTANT
_____
_____
_____

Date: _____ Patient name: _____
APPOINTMENT: _____

## Patient Details
_____
_____
_____
_____

## Patient History
_____
_____
_____
_____

| SYMPTOMS | MEDICATION | CONCERNS |
|---|---|---|
|  |  |  |

## My Thoughts and Notes
_____
_____
_____
_____

## Future Check Up/s
_____
_____
_____

### IMPORTANT
_____
_____

**Date:** _____  **Patient name:** _____

APPOINTMENT: _____

*Patient Details*

_____
_____
_____
_____

*Patient History*

_____
_____
_____
_____

| SYMPTOMS | MEDICATION | CONCERNS |
|----------|------------|----------|
|          |            |          |

*My Thoughts and Notes* | *Future Check Up/s*

IMPORTANT

Date: _____ Patient name: _____

APPOINTMENT: _____

Patient Details
_____
_____
_____
_____

Patient History
_____
_____
_____
_____
_____

SYMPTOMS        MEDICATION        CONCERNS

My Thoughts and Notes                Future Check Up/s
_____    _____
_____    _____
_____    _____
_____    _____
_____
_____

IMPORTANT
_____
_____
_____

Date: _____ Patient name: _____

APPOINTMENT: _____

## Patient Details
_____
_____
_____
_____

## Patient History
_____
_____
_____
_____
_____

| SYMPTOMS | MEDICATION | CONCERNS |
|---|---|---|
|  |  |  |

## My thoughts and Notes | ## Future Check Up/s

_____ | _____
_____ | _____
_____ | _____
_____ | _____

IMPORTANT
_____
_____
_____

# Date: _____  Patient name: _____

APPOINTMENT: _____

## Patient Details
_____
_____
_____
_____

## Patient History
_____
_____
_____
_____
_____

| SYMPTOMS | MEDICATION | CONCERNS |
|---|---|---|
|  |  |  |

## My Thoughts and Notes

## Future Check Up/s
_____
_____
_____
_____

_____
_____
_____
_____
_____

## IMPORTANT
_____
_____
_____

Date: _____  Patient name: _____

APPOINTMENT: _____

## Patient Details

_____
_____
_____
_____

## Patient History

_____
_____
_____
_____

| SYMPTOMS | MEDICATION | CONCERNS |
|---|---|---|
|  |  |  |

### My Thoughts and Notes

_____
_____
_____
_____

### Future Check Up/s

_____
_____
_____

### IMPORTANT

_____
_____

*Date:* _____  *Patient name:* _____

APPOINTMENT: _____

*Patient Details*
_____
_____
_____
_____

*Patient History*
_____
_____
_____
_____
_____

| SYMPTOMS | MEDICATION | CONCERNS |
|---|---|---|
|  |  |  |

*My Thoughts and Notes*                *Future Check Up/s*
_____         _____
_____         _____
_____         _____
_____         _____
_____
_____
_____

IMPORTANT
_____
_____
_____

Date: _____  Patient name: _____

APPOINTMENT: _____

## Patient Details
_____
_____
_____
_____

## Patient History
_____
_____
_____
_____

| SYMPTOMS | MEDICATION | CONCERNS |
|---|---|---|
|  |  |  |

## My thoughts and Notes
_____
_____
_____
_____
_____

## Future Check Up's
_____
_____
_____

IMPORTANT

Date: _____ Patient name: _____

APPOINTMENT: _____

Patient Details
_____
_____
_____
_____

Patient History
_____
_____
_____
_____

| SYMPTOMS | MEDICATION | CONCERNS |
|---|---|---|
|  |  |  |

My Thoughts and Notes

Future Check Up/s
_____
_____
_____
_____

IMPORTANT
_____
_____

# Date: _____  Patient name: _____

APPOINTMENT: _____

## Patient Details
_____
_____
_____
_____

## Patient History
_____
_____
_____
_____

| SYMPTOMS | MEDICATION | CONCERNS |
|---|---|---|
|  |  |  |

## My thoughts and Notes

_____
_____
_____
_____
_____

## Future Check Up/s

_____
_____
_____

### IMPORTANT
_____
_____

Date: _____ Patient name: _____

APPOINTMENT: _____

## Patient Details
_____
_____
_____
_____

## Patient History
_____
_____
_____
_____
_____

| SYMPTOMS | MEDICATION | CONCERNS |
|---|---|---|
| | | |

## My Thoughts and Notes / Future Check Up/s

_____  _____
_____  _____
_____  _____
_____
_____
_____

IMPORTANT

_____
_____

# Date: _____  Patient name: _____

APPOINTMENT: _____

## Patient Details
_____
_____
_____
_____

## Patient History
_____
_____
_____
_____

| SYMPTOMS | MEDICATION | CONCERNS |
|---|---|---|
|  |  |  |

## My thoughts and Notes
_____
_____
_____
_____

## Future Check Up/s
_____
_____
_____

## IMPORTANT
_____
_____
_____

Date: _____  Patient name: _____

APPOINTMENT: _____

## Patient Details
_____
_____
_____
_____

## Patient History
_____
_____
_____
_____

| SYMPTOMS | MEDICATION | CONCERNS |
|----------|------------|----------|
|          |            |          |

### My Thoughts and Notes
_____
_____
_____
_____

### Future Check Up/s
_____
_____
_____

### IMPORTANT
_____
_____
_____

Date: _____ Patient name: _____

APPOINTMENT: _____

## Patient Details

_____
_____
_____
_____

## Patient History

_____
_____
_____
_____

| SYMPTOMS | MEDICATION | CONCERNS |
|---|---|---|
|  |  |  |

## My Thoughts and Notes / Future Check Up/s

_____
_____
_____
_____

IMPORTANT

Date: _____  Patient name: _____

APPOINTMENT: _____

## Patient Details
_____
_____
_____
_____

## Patient History
_____
_____
_____
_____
_____

| SYMPTOMS | MEDICATION | CONCERNS |
|---|---|---|
|  |  |  |

### My Thoughts and Notes                    ### Future Check Up/s
_____    _____
_____    _____
_____    _____
_____
_____
_____
_____

IMPORTANT

Date: _____  Patient name: _____

APPOINTMENT: _____

## Patient Details
_____
_____
_____
_____

## Patient History
_____
_____
_____
_____

| SYMPTOMS | MEDICATION | CONCERNS |
|---|---|---|
|  |  |  |

### My Thoughts and Notes
_____
_____
_____
_____

### Future Check Up/s
_____
_____

IMPORTANT

Date: _____ Patient name: _____

APPOINTMENT: _____

## Patient Details

_____
_____
_____
_____

## Patient History

_____
_____
_____
_____
_____

| SYMPTOMS | MEDICATION | CONCERNS |
|---|---|---|
|  |  |  |

### My Thoughts and Notes

_____
_____
_____
_____
_____
_____

### Future Check Up/s

_____
_____
_____
_____

IMPORTANT

_____
_____
_____

**Date:** _____  **Patient name:** _____

APPOINTMENT: _____

*Patient Details*

_____
_____
_____
_____

*Patient History*

_____
_____
_____
_____

| SYMPTOMS | MEDICATION | CONCERNS |
|----------|------------|----------|
|          |            |          |

*My Thoughts and Notes*                *Future Check Up/s*

IMPORTANT

Date: _____  Patient name: _____

APPOINTMENT: _____

## Patient Details
_____
_____
_____
_____

## Patient History
_____
_____
_____
_____

| SYMPTOMS | MEDICATION | CONCERNS |
|---|---|---|
|  |  |  |

### My Thoughts and Notes
_____
_____
_____
_____
_____

### Future Check Up/s
_____
_____
_____

IMPORTANT
_____
_____
_____

**Date:** _____  **Patient name:** _____

APPOINTMENT: _____

### Patient Details

_____
_____
_____
_____

### Patient History

_____
_____
_____
_____

| SYMPTOMS | MEDICATION | CONCERNS |
|---|---|---|
|  |  |  |

### My Thoughts and Notes

_____
_____
_____
_____

### Future Check Up/s

_____
_____
_____

IMPORTANT
_____
_____

Date: _____ Patient name: _____
APPOINTMENT: _____

## Patient Details
_____
_____
_____
_____

## Patient History
_____
_____
_____
_____

| SYMPTOMS | MEDICATION | CONCERNS |
|----------|------------|----------|
|          |            |          |

### My Thoughts and Notes
_____
_____
_____
_____
_____

### Future Check Up's
_____
_____
_____

IMPORTANT
_____
_____

# Date: _____  Patient name: _____

APPOINTMENT: _____

## Patient Details
_____
_____
_____
_____

## Patient History
_____
_____
_____
_____

| SYMPTOMS | MEDICATION | CONCERNS |
|---|---|---|
| | | |

### My Thoughts and Notes
_____
_____
_____
_____
_____

### Future Check Up/s
_____
_____
_____

### IMPORTANT
_____
_____

**Date:** _____  **Patient name:** _____

APPOINTMENT: _____

*Patient Details*
_____
_____
_____
_____

*Patient History*
_____
_____
_____
_____

| SYMPTOMS | MEDICATION | CONCERNS |
|----------|------------|----------|
|          |            |          |

*My Thoughts and Notes*     *Future Check Up/s*

IMPORTANT

Date: _____  Patient name: _____
APPOINTMENT: _____

## Patient Details
_____
_____
_____
_____

## Patient History
_____
_____
_____
_____

| SYMPTOMS | MEDICATION | CONCERNS |
|---|---|---|
|  |  |  |

## My Thoughts and Notes
_____
_____
_____
_____

## Future Check Up/s
_____
_____

IMPORTANT
_____
_____

Date: _____   Patient name: _____
APPOINTMENT: _____

## Patient Details
_____
_____
_____
_____

## Patient History
_____
_____
_____
_____

| SYMPTOMS | MEDICATION | CONCERNS |
|---|---|---|
|  |  |  |

## My Thoughts and Notes
_____
_____
_____
_____
_____

## Future Check Up/s
_____
_____
_____

IMPORTANT
_____
_____
_____

Date: _____ Patient name: _____
APPOINTMENT: _____

### Patient Details
_____
_____
_____
_____

### Patient History
_____
_____
_____
_____

| SYMPTOMS | MEDICATION | CONCERNS |
|---|---|---|
|  |  |  |

### My thoughts and Notes
_____
_____
_____
_____

### Future Check Up's
_____
_____

IMPORTANT
_____
_____

Date: _____  Patient name: _____

APPOINTMENT: _____

## Patient Details
_____
_____
_____
_____

## Patient History
_____
_____
_____
_____

| SYMPTOMS | MEDICATION | CONCERNS |
|---|---|---|
|  |  |  |

### My Thoughts and Notes
_____
_____
_____
_____
_____

### Future Check Up's
_____
_____
_____

IMPORTANT
_____
_____

Date: _____  Patient name: _____

APPOINTMENT: _____

## Patient Details
_____
_____
_____
_____

## Patient History
_____
_____
_____
_____
_____

| SYMPTOMS | MEDICATION | CONCERNS |
|----------|------------|----------|
|          |            |          |

## My Thoughts and Notes
_____
_____
_____
_____
_____

## Future Check Up/s
_____
_____
_____

IMPORTANT
_____
_____

**Date:** _____  **Patient name:** _____

APPOINTMENT: _____

## Patient Details

_____
_____
_____
_____

## Patient History

_____
_____
_____
_____

| SYMPTOMS | MEDICATION | CONCERNS |
|---|---|---|
|   |   |   |

### My thoughts and Notes

_____
_____
_____
_____
_____

### Future Check Up/s

_____
_____
_____

IMPORTANT

_____
_____

Date: _____  Patient name: _____
APPOINTMENT: _____

## Patient Details
_____
_____
_____
_____

## Patient History
_____
_____
_____
_____

| SYMPTOMS | MEDICATION | CONCERNS |
|---|---|---|
|  |  |  |

## My thoughts and Notes
_____
_____
_____
_____
_____

## Future Check Up/s
_____
_____
_____

IMPORTANT
_____
_____
_____

Date: _____ Patient name: _____

APPOINTMENT: _____

## Patient Details
_____
_____
_____
_____

## Patient History
_____
_____
_____
_____

| SYMPTOMS | MEDICATION | CONCERNS |
|---|---|---|
|  |  |  |

## My Thoughts and Notes

## Future Check Up/s

_____
_____
_____
_____
_____

IMPORTANT
_____
_____

Date: _____  Patient name: _____

APPOINTMENT: _____

## Patient Details

_____
_____
_____
_____

## Patient History

_____
_____
_____
_____
_____

| SYMPTOMS | MEDICATION | CONCERNS |
|---|---|---|
|  |  |  |

### My Thoughts and Notes

### Future Check Up/s

IMPORTANT

Date: _____  Patient name: _____

APPOINTMENT: _____

## Patient Details
_____
_____
_____
_____

## Patient History
_____
_____
_____
_____
_____

| SYMPTOMS | MEDICATION | CONCERNS |
|---|---|---|
|  |  |  |

### My Thoughts and Notes
_____
_____
_____
_____
_____

### Future Check Up's
_____
_____
_____

IMPORTANT
_____
_____
_____

Date: _____  Patient name: _____

APPOINTMENT: _____

## Patient Details
_____
_____
_____
_____

## Patient History
_____
_____
_____
_____
_____

| SYMPTOMS | MEDICATION | CONCERNS |
|---|---|---|
|  |  |  |

## My Thoughts and Notes
_____
_____
_____
_____
_____

## Future Check Up/s
_____
_____
_____

IMPORTANT
_____
_____

Date: _____    Patient name: _____
APPOINTMENT: _____

## Patient Details
_____
_____
_____
_____

## Patient History
_____
_____
_____
_____

| SYMPTOMS | MEDICATION | CONCERNS |
|---|---|---|
|  |  |  |

## My Thoughts and Notes
_____
_____
_____
_____

## Future Check Up/s
_____
_____

IMPORTANT
_____
_____

Date: _____  Patient name: _____

APPOINTMENT: _____

## Patient Details
_____
_____
_____
_____

## Patient History
_____
_____
_____
_____

| SYMPTOMS | MEDICATION | CONCERNS |
|---|---|---|
|  |  |  |

## My Thoughts and Notes / Future Check Up/s

_____
_____
_____
_____

IMPORTANT

_____
_____
_____

Date: _____  Patient name: _____

APPOINTMENT: _____

## Patient Details
_____
_____
_____
_____

## Patient History
_____
_____
_____
_____

| SYMPTOMS | MEDICATION | CONCERNS |
|----------|------------|----------|
|          |            |          |

## My Thoughts and Notes
_____
_____
_____
_____
_____

## Future Check Up's
_____
_____
_____

IMPORTANT
_____
_____

Date: _____ Patient name: _____

APPOINTMENT: _____

## Patient Details

_____
_____
_____
_____

## Patient History

_____
_____
_____
_____

| SYMPTOMS | MEDICATION | CONCERNS |
|---|---|---|
|  |  |  |

### My thoughts and Notes

_____
_____
_____
_____
_____

### Future Check Up/s

_____
_____
_____

IMPORTANT

_____
_____
_____

Date: _____ Patient name: _____
APPOINTMENT: _____

## Patient Details
_____
_____
_____
_____

## Patient History
_____
_____
_____
_____

| SYMPTOMS | MEDICATION | CONCERNS |
|---|---|---|
|  |  |  |

## My Thoughts and Notes
## Future Check Up/s

_____  _____
_____  _____
_____  _____
_____
_____
_____

IMPORTANT
_____
_____

Date: _____  Patient name: _____
APPOINTMENT: _____

Patient Details
_____
_____
_____
_____

Patient History
_____
_____
_____
_____

SYMPTOMS  MEDICATION  CONCERNS

My Thoughts and Notes   Future Check Up/s
_____
_____
_____
_____
_____

IMPORTANT
_____
_____

**Date:** _____ **Patient name:** _____

APPOINTMENT: _____

## Patient Details

_____
_____
_____
_____

## Patient History

_____
_____
_____
_____

| SYMPTOMS | MEDICATION | CONCERNS |
|---|---|---|
|  |  |  |

### My thoughts and Notes

_____
_____
_____
_____

### Future Check Up/s

_____
_____

IMPORTANT

_____
_____
_____

*Date:* _____  *Patient name:* _____

APPOINTMENT: _____

*Patient Details*
_____
_____
_____
_____

*Patient History*
_____
_____
_____
_____

| SYMPTOMS | MEDICATION | CONCERNS |
|---|---|---|
|  |  |  |

*My Thoughts and Notes*     *Future Check Up/s*
_____     _____
_____     _____
_____     _____
_____
_____

IMPORTANT
_____
_____
_____

# Date: _____  Patient name: _____

APPOINTMENT: _____

## Patient Details
_____
_____
_____
_____

## Patient History
_____
_____
_____
_____

| SYMPTOMS | MEDICATION | CONCERNS |
|---|---|---|
|  |  |  |

## My Thoughts and Notes
_____
_____
_____
_____
_____

## Future Check Up's
_____
_____
_____

## IMPORTANT
_____
_____
_____

Date: _____  Patient name: _____

APPOINTMENT: _____

## Patient Details
_____
_____
_____
_____

## Patient History
_____
_____
_____
_____

| SYMPTOMS | MEDICATION | CONCERNS |
|---|---|---|
|  |  |  |

## My Thoughts and Notes
_____
_____
_____
_____
_____

## Future Check Up/s
_____
_____
_____

IMPORTANT

Date: _____  Patient name: _____

APPOINTMENT: _____

## Patient Details

_____
_____
_____
_____

## Patient History

_____
_____
_____
_____
_____

| SYMPTOMS | MEDICATION | CONCERNS |
|---|---|---|
|  |  |  |

## My thoughts and Notes

## Future Check Up/s

_____
_____
_____
_____
_____

IMPORTANT

_____
_____

Date: _____  Patient name: _____

APPOINTMENT: _____

## Patient Details

_____
_____
_____
_____

## Patient History

_____
_____
_____
_____

| SYMPTOMS | MEDICATION | CONCERNS |
|---|---|---|
|  |  |  |

## My Thoughts and Notes

## Future Check Up/s

_____
_____
_____
_____

IMPORTANT

Date: _____  Patient name: _____

APPOINTMENT: _____

## Patient Details
_____
_____
_____
_____

## Patient History
_____
_____
_____
_____

| SYMPTOMS | MEDICATION | CONCERNS |
|---|---|---|
|  |  |  |

## My Thoughts and Notes
_____
_____
_____
_____
_____

## Future Check Up/s
_____
_____
_____

IMPORTANT
_____
_____

Date: _____ Patient name: _____
APPOINTMENT: _____

## Patient Details
_____
_____
_____
_____

## Patient History
_____
_____
_____
_____

| SYMPTOMS | MEDICATION | CONCERNS |
|---|---|---|
|  |  |  |

## My Thoughts and Notes
_____
_____
_____
_____

## Future Check Up's
_____
_____
_____

IMPORTANT
_____
_____

Date: _____ Patient name: _____

APPOINTMENT: _____

## Patient Details
_____
_____
_____
_____

## Patient History
_____
_____
_____
_____

| SYMPTOMS | MEDICATION | CONCERNS |
|---|---|---|
| | | |

## My Thoughts and Notes
_____
_____
_____
_____
_____

## Future Check Up's
_____
_____
_____

IMPORTANT
_____
_____

Date: _____  Patient name: _____

APPOINTMENT: _____

## Patient Details
_____
_____
_____
_____

## Patient History
_____
_____
_____
_____

| SYMPTOMS | MEDICATION | CONCERNS |
|---|---|---|
|  |  |  |

## My Thoughts and Notes
_____
_____
_____
_____

## Future Check Up/s
_____
_____

IMPORTANT
_____
_____

Date: _____ Patient name: _____
APPOINTMENT: _____

## Patient Details
_____
_____
_____
_____

## Patient History
_____
_____
_____
_____

| SYMPTOMS | MEDICATION | CONCERNS |
|----------|------------|----------|
|          |            |          |

### My Thoughts and Notes
_____
_____
_____
_____
_____

### Future Check Up/s
_____
_____
_____

IMPORTANT
_____
_____
_____

Date: _____  Patient name: _____

APPOINTMENT: _____

Patient Details
_____
_____
_____
_____

Patient History
_____
_____
_____
_____
_____

| SYMPTOMS | MEDICATION | CONCERNS |
|---|---|---|
|  |  |  |

My Thoughts and Notes
_____
_____
_____
_____
_____
_____

Future Check Up/s
_____
_____
_____

IMPORTANT
_____
_____
_____

*Date:* _____   *Patient name:* _____

APPOINTMENT: _____

*Patient Details*

_____
_____
_____
_____

*Patient History*

_____
_____
_____
_____
_____

| SYMPTOMS | MEDICATION | CONCERNS |
|---|---|---|
|  |  |  |

*My Thoughts and Notes*                *Future Check Up/s*

_____          _____
_____          _____
_____          _____
_____
_____
_____

IMPORTANT

_____
_____
_____

Date: _____ Patient name: _____
APPOINTMENT: _____

## Patient Details
_____
_____
_____
_____

## Patient History
_____
_____
_____
_____

| SYMPTOMS | MEDICATION | CONCERNS |
|---|---|---|
|  |  |  |

## My Thoughts and Notes
_____
_____
_____
_____
_____

## Future Check Up/s
_____
_____
_____

IMPORTANT
_____
_____

**Date:** _____  **Patient name:** _____

APPOINTMENT: _____

*Patient Details*
_____
_____
_____
_____

*Patient History*
_____
_____
_____
_____

| SYMPTOMS | MEDICATION | CONCERNS |
|---|---|---|
|  |  |  |

*My thoughts and Notes*                    *Future Check Up/s*
_____    _____
_____    _____
_____    _____
_____
_____
_____

IMPORTANT
_____
_____

**Date:** _____ **Patient name:** _____

APPOINTMENT: _____

## Patient Details

_____
_____
_____
_____

## Patient History

_____
_____
_____
_____

| SYMPTOMS | MEDICATION | CONCERNS |
|----------|------------|----------|
|          |            |          |

## My Thoughts and Notes

_____
_____
_____
_____

## Future Check Up/s

_____
_____

IMPORTANT
_____
_____
_____

*Date:* _____  *Patient name:* _____

APPOINTMENT: _____

*Patient Details*

_____
_____
_____
_____

*Patient History*

_____
_____
_____
_____

| SYMPTOMS | MEDICATION | CONCERNS |
|---|---|---|
|  |  |  |

*My Thoughts and Notes*                *Future Check Up's*

IMPORTANT

Date: _____ Patient name: _____
APPOINTMENT: _____

## Patient Details
_____
_____
_____
_____

## Patient History
_____
_____
_____
_____

| SYMPTOMS | MEDICATION | CONCERNS |
|---|---|---|
|  |  |  |

## My Thoughts and Notes
_____
_____
_____
_____
_____

### Future Check Up/s
_____
_____
_____

IMPORTANT
_____
_____

Date: _____ Patient name: _____

APPOINTMENT: _____

## Patient Details
_____
_____
_____
_____

## Patient History
_____
_____
_____
_____

| SYMPTOMS | MEDICATION | CONCERNS |
|---|---|---|
|  |  |  |

## My Thoughts and Notes
_____
_____
_____
_____
_____

## Future Check Up's
_____
_____
_____

IMPORTANT
_____
_____
_____

Date: _____ Patient name: _____
APPOINTMENT: _____

## Patient Details
_____
_____
_____
_____
_____

## Patient History
_____
_____
_____
_____
_____

| SYMPTOMS | MEDICATION | CONCERNS |
|---|---|---|
|  |  |  |

## My Thoughts and Notes
_____
_____
_____
_____
_____

## Future Check Up/s
_____
_____
_____

IMPORTANT

Date: _____  Patient name: _____

APPOINTMENT: _____

## Patient Details
_____
_____
_____
_____

## Patient History
_____
_____
_____
_____

| SYMPTOMS | MEDICATION | CONCERNS |
|---|---|---|
|  |  |  |

### My thoughts and Notes
_____
_____
_____
_____
_____

### Future Check Up's
_____
_____

IMPORTANT
_____
_____

# Date: _____  Patient name: _____

APPOINTMENT: _____

## Patient Details
_____
_____
_____
_____

## Patient History
_____
_____
_____
_____

| SYMPTOMS | MEDICATION | CONCERNS |
|---|---|---|
|  |  |  |

## My Thoughts and Notes
_____
_____
_____
_____

## Future Check Up/s
_____
_____

IMPORTANT
_____
_____

# Date: _____ Patient name: _____

APPOINTMENT: _____

## Patient Details
_____
_____
_____
_____

## Patient History
_____
_____
_____
_____
_____

| SYMPTOMS | MEDICATION | CONCERNS |
|---|---|---|
|  |  |  |

### My thoughts and Notes / Future Check Up/s

_____
_____
_____
_____
_____

### IMPORTANT
_____
_____
_____

# Date: _____  Patient name: _____

APPOINTMENT: _____

## Patient Details
_____
_____
_____
_____

## Patient History
_____
_____
_____
_____

| SYMPTOMS | MEDICATION | CONCERNS |
|---|---|---|
|  |  |  |

## My thoughts and Notes
_____
_____
_____
_____

## Future Check Up's
_____
_____

IMPORTANT
_____
_____

**Date:** _____  **Patient name:** _____

APPOINTMENT: _____

## Patient Details
_____
_____
_____
_____

## Patient History
_____
_____
_____
_____

| SYMPTOMS | MEDICATION | CONCERNS |
|----------|------------|----------|
|          |            |          |

### My thoughts and Notes
_____
_____
_____
_____
_____

### Future Check Up/s
_____
_____
_____

IMPORTANT
_____
_____

Date: _____ Patient name: _____

APPOINTMENT: _____

## Patient Details
_____
_____
_____
_____

## Patient History
_____
_____
_____
_____

| SYMPTOMS | MEDICATION | CONCERNS |
|---|---|---|
|  |  |  |

## My Thoughts and Notes | Future Check Up/s

_____
_____
_____
_____
_____
_____

IMPORTANT

_____
_____

Date: _____  Patient name: _____
APPOINTMENT: _____

## Patient Details
_____
_____
_____
_____

## Patient History
_____
_____
_____
_____

| SYMPTOMS | MEDICATION | CONCERNS |
|---|---|---|
|  |  |  |

## My Thoughts and Notes
_____
_____
_____
_____
_____
_____

## Future Check Up/s
_____
_____
_____

## IMPORTANT
_____
_____
_____

Date: _____ Patient name: _____
APPOINTMENT: _____

## Patient Details
_____
_____
_____
_____

## Patient History
_____
_____
_____
_____

| SYMPTOMS | MEDICATION | CONCERNS |
|---|---|---|
|  |  |  |

## My Thoughts and Notes
_____
_____
_____
_____
_____

## Future Check Up/s
_____
_____
_____

IMPORTANT

Date: _____  Patient name: _____

APPOINTMENT: _____

## Patient Details

_____
_____
_____
_____
_____

## Patient History

_____
_____
_____
_____
_____

| SYMPTOMS | MEDICATION | CONCERNS |
|---|---|---|
|  |  |  |

### My Thoughts and Notes

_____
_____
_____
_____
_____
_____

### Future Check Up/s

_____
_____
_____

IMPORTANT

_____
_____

Date: _____ Patient name: _____

APPOINTMENT: _____

## Patient Details

_____
_____
_____
_____

## Patient History

_____
_____
_____
_____
_____

| SYMPTOMS | MEDICATION | CONCERNS |
|---|---|---|
|  |  |  |

### My Thoughts and Notes

### Future Check Up/s

_____
_____
_____
_____
_____

IMPORTANT

_____
_____

Date: _____  Patient name: _____

APPOINTMENT: _____

## Patient Details
_____
_____
_____
_____

## Patient History
_____
_____
_____
_____

| SYMPTOMS | MEDICATION | CONCERNS |
|---|---|---|
|  |  |  |

## My Thoughts and Notes
_____
_____
_____
_____
_____

## Future Check Up/s
_____
_____
_____

IMPORTANT
_____
_____
_____

# Date: _____  Patient name: _____

APPOINTMENT: _____

## Patient Details
_____
_____
_____
_____

## Patient History
_____
_____
_____
_____

| SYMPTOMS | MEDICATION | CONCERNS |
|---|---|---|
|  |  |  |

## My Thoughts and Notes
_____
_____
_____
_____
_____

## Future Check Up/s
_____
_____

IMPORTANT
_____
_____
_____

Made in the USA
Las Vegas, NV
31 March 2025